Table of contents

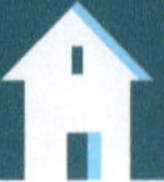

This book is only to help you learn. It should not be used to replace any advice or treatment from a nurse or doctor.

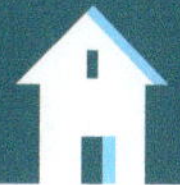

This booklet is to help you get ready to care for a weak or disabled person at home. You can learn how to prepare your house and make it safe for your loved one. You will find tips from experts and drawings and instructions to help you make a plan for your home. Having a plan can give you peace of mind. And with your mind at ease, you will be freer to enjoy and care for your loved one.

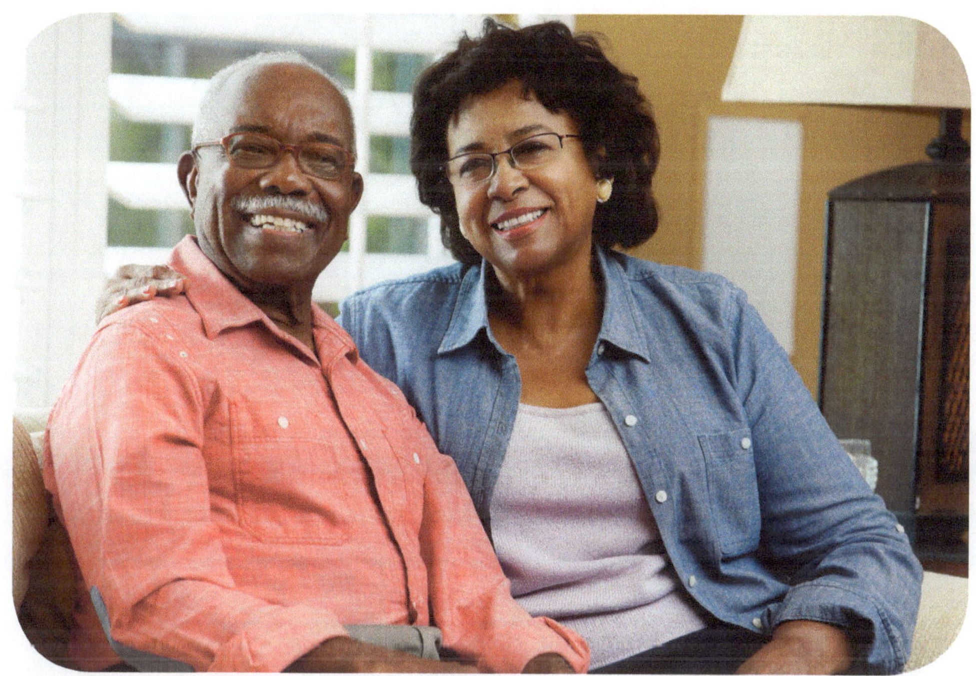

If you are feeling a little overwhelmed by your loved one coming home, relax a little. Being a care giver may be a new role for you, and no one expects you to be perfect. Your loved one's health team is just a phone call away. Call them when you need help or advice. And if friends offer to give you a break, let them. When you are relaxed, your loved one feels it.

We do not intend to be sexist, but to keep the text simple, we have used "he" and "him" throughout when talking about your loved one.

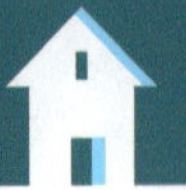

You are now a big part of your loved one's health team. Others on the team will also help you. Some of these health team members are:

- **Registered Nurse (RN)**– gives and teaches you how to give nursing care. Plans care and can help get PT, OT and social worker involved.

- **Social Worker (SW)**– gives emotional support and financial guidance; tells about community services and financial aid.

- **Occupational Therapist (OT)**– teaches self-care skills (bathing, grooming, eating, dressing, etc.) and visual-perceptual skills (how the brain interprets what the eyes see). Can tell you about special equipment and where to get it.

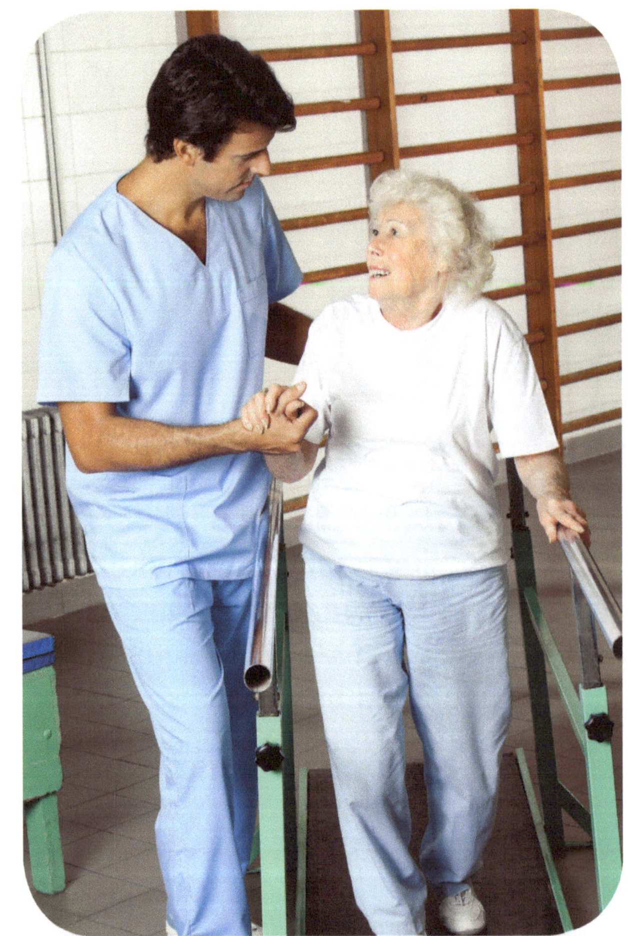

- **Physical Therapist (PT)**– teaches skills for moving safely, relearning how to walk or using a wheelchair. Can tell you about wheelchairs, walkers, etc. and where to get them.

These health team members can give services through your home health agency. If you do not have a home health service, ask your doctor about getting one.

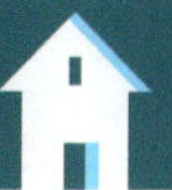

The first part of getting someone settled at home is to help him get from the car to the door safely and without a big effort on his part or yours. Use the checklist on page 21 to note changes you need to make.

Parking

Park the car as close to the house as you can. If you park in a garage, make sure there is enough room for the person to get in and out of the car with the door open all the way. If a wheelchair or walker is used, allow enough room for that, too.

Walkways and Doors

Check the surface your loved one will cross from the car to the house. If it's grass, keep it cut short. Pushing a wheelchair over dirt and stones can be hard. Measure the width of the walkway and the garage and house doors to make sure there is room for a walker or wheelchair. Measure the wheelchair at its widest point and allow room for fingers. If there are steps, you may need to add a ramp. Read the next page for ramp guidelines.

The PT can answer your questions and give advice on any of this if you need it.

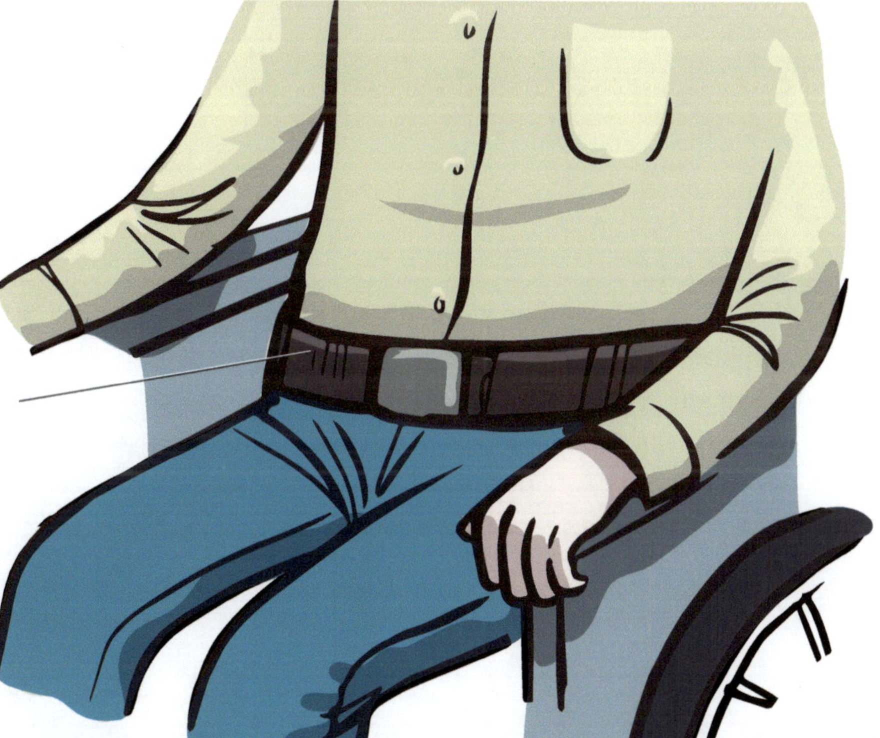

Always wear seatbelt on rough ground.

How to build a ramp

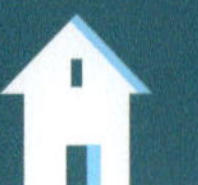

To make sure your ramp plan will work for your family member, review it with the physical therapist.

1. For every inch of rise (the height of the steps plus the door threshold), you need 1 foot of ramp. The rise shown here is 24 inches, the ramp length is 24 feet.

2. Make the ramp 42 inches wide, and use pressure-treated lumber, marine plywood or concrete. Make the surface nonskid (gritty paper adhesive, nonskid paint or, if concrete, a broom finish which has been swept from side to side, not up and down).

3. Build a 5 foot x 5 foot platform even with the door threshold. Make sure there is **at least** an 18 inch space when door is open all the way for wheelchair to approach door.

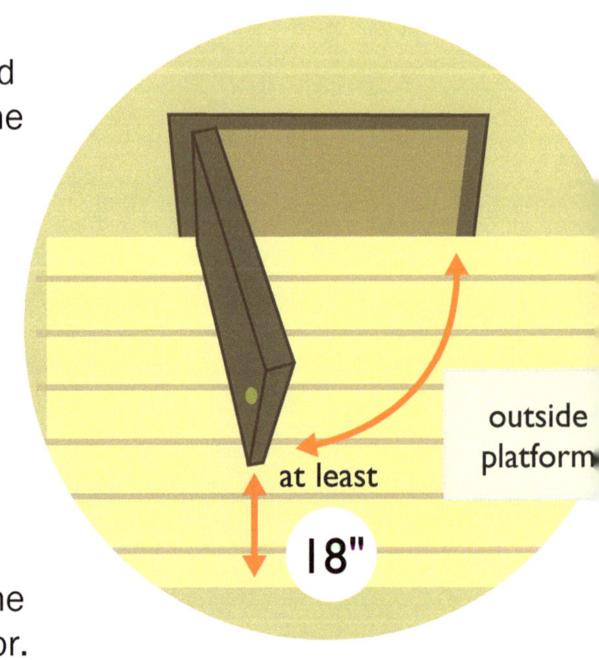

Hint:

You can buy nonskid paint or make your own by mixing sand with the paint. Use 1 pound silica sand for each gallon of paint.

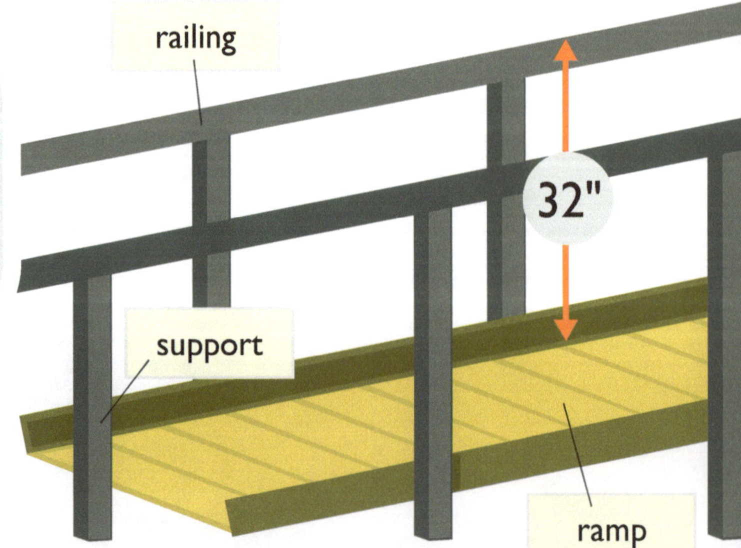

4. Put railings on both sides, not more than 32 inches high. Railings should be 1½ inches thick, extend 1 to 1½ feet beyond ramp and, for safety, have a turned down end.

5. Put a 4 inch high curb along both sides of ramp and platform so wheelchair, crutches or walker tips can't slip over sides.

6. Ramps that turn or are longer than 30 feet need more platforms for resting and so that the wheelchair can't build up too much speed.

Hint:
You can also buy ramp "kits". Check on-line for more information.

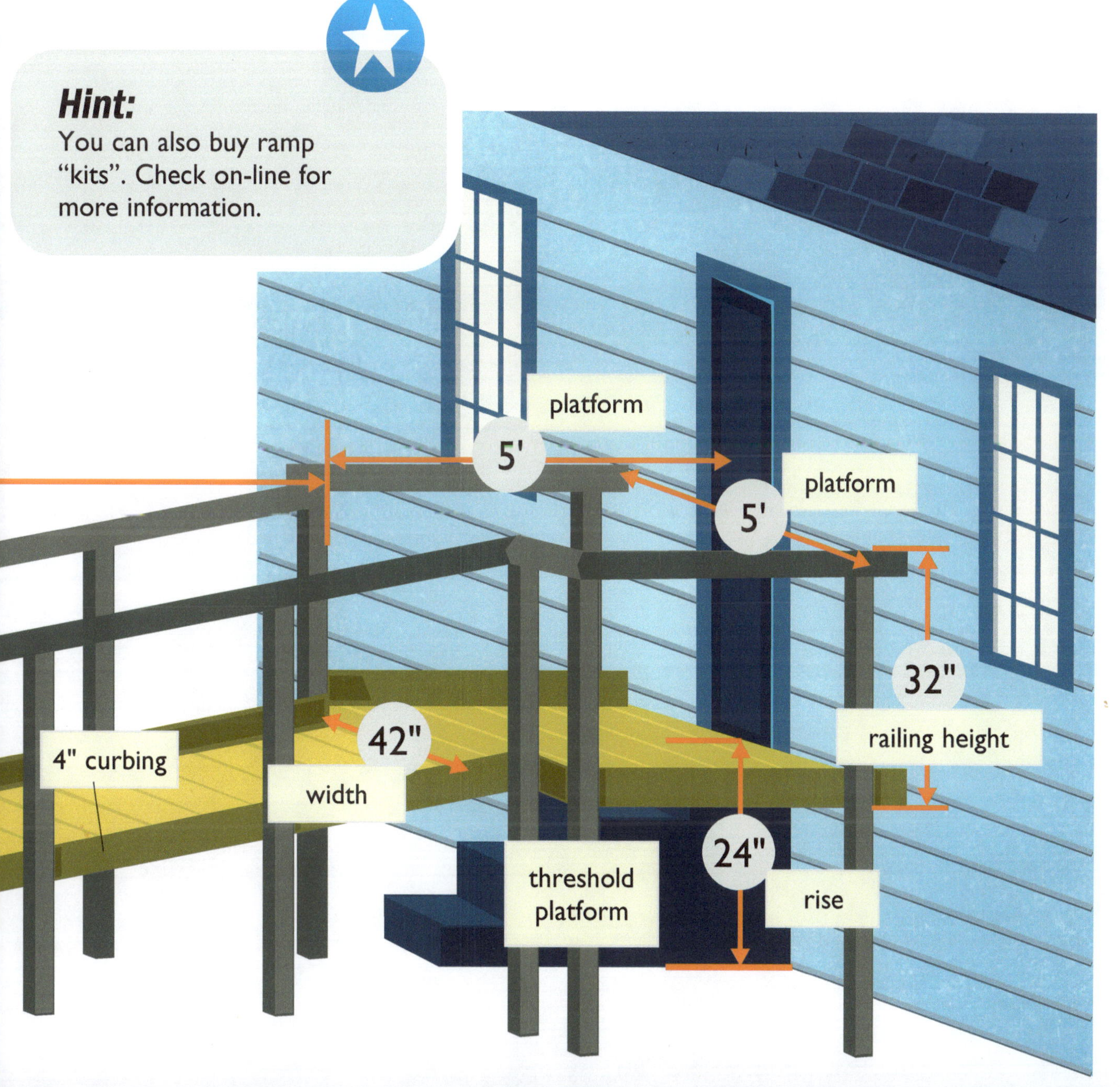

Handrails

Add handrails along both sides of steps, walkways and ramps. For safety, extend handrails beyond top and bottom of ramps and steps.

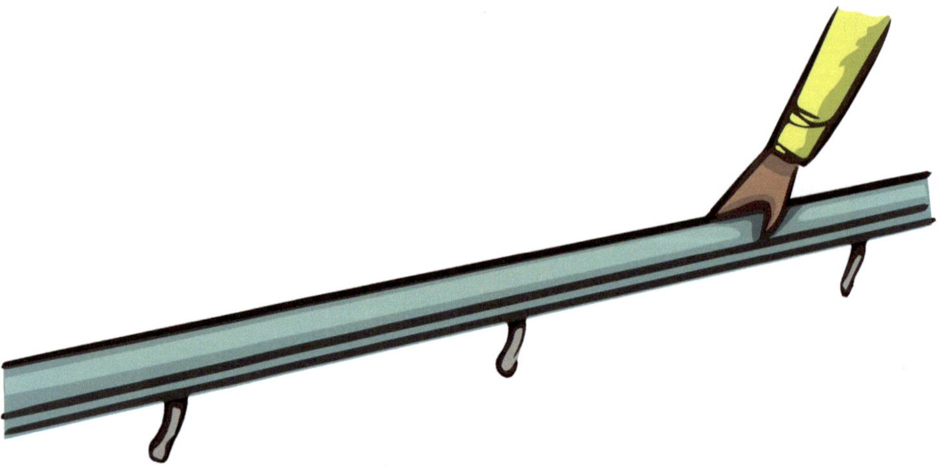

Lighting

Make sure your garage, entries to the house, walkways and ramps are well lit. You should be able to see well, with no glare from lights and no shadows. These can cause accidents.

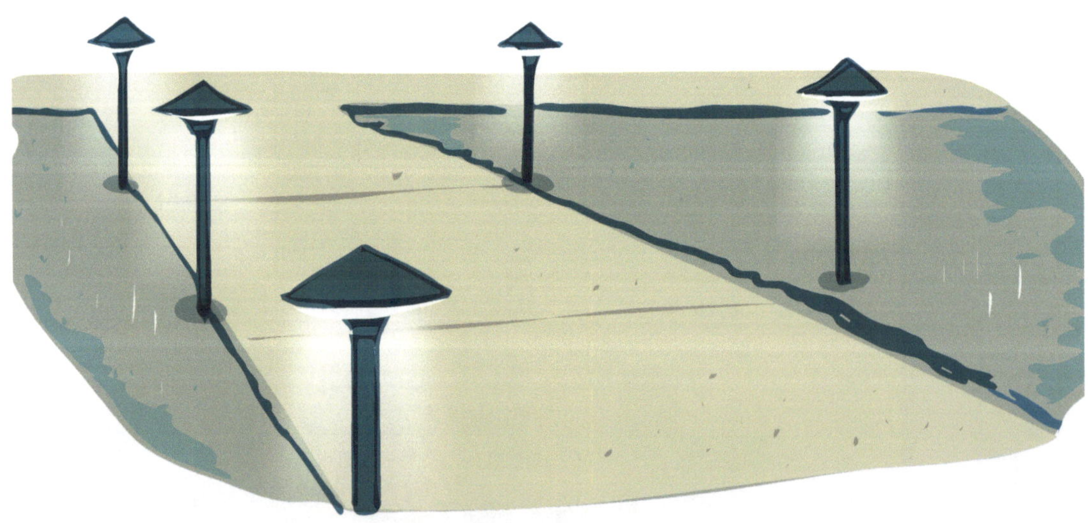

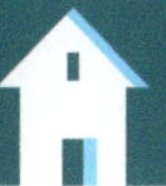

Now that you've checked the outside of your house, you get the idea about the kinds of changes that can help your family member. Do the same thing on the inside, and note any changes needed on the checklist on page 22. Think about the things your loved one will do in each room and what you can change to make it easier for him.

Floors

Waxed floors and thick carpet can be hard and even dangerous for someone who has a problem walking or must use a walker, cane or wheelchair. It's best to get rid of throw rugs. These kinds of floors would work better:

- nonskid surface

- short-pile carpet

- indoor/outdoor carpet

Also, keep floors clear of toys, shoes or other objects. If you have to walk around cords or wires, move items or have an electrician install another outlet.

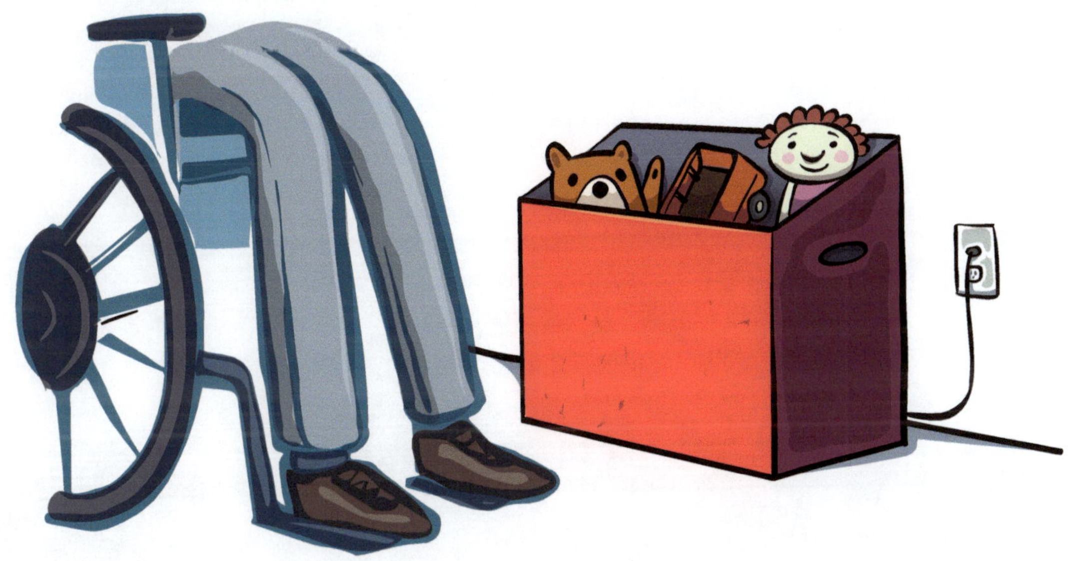

Furniture

Make enough room between furniture so your loved one can move around with ease. A 5 foot x 5 foot space to move and turn around is best. Cover any sharp edges on furniture that could catch on a crutch, cane, walker or wheelchair.

Stairs

If the person can use stairs, make sure there are sturdy handrails on both sides. If there is no handrail, you may need to install one. Make sure the handrails are as long as the stairs. Strips of orange or yellow tape on the edge of the stairs can help someone with poor vision. If the person's vision is very poor, a gate across the top of the stairs can help avoid an accident.

If your loved one has to stay on one floor, make sure his room is on the same floor as the bathroom and kitchen or dining room.

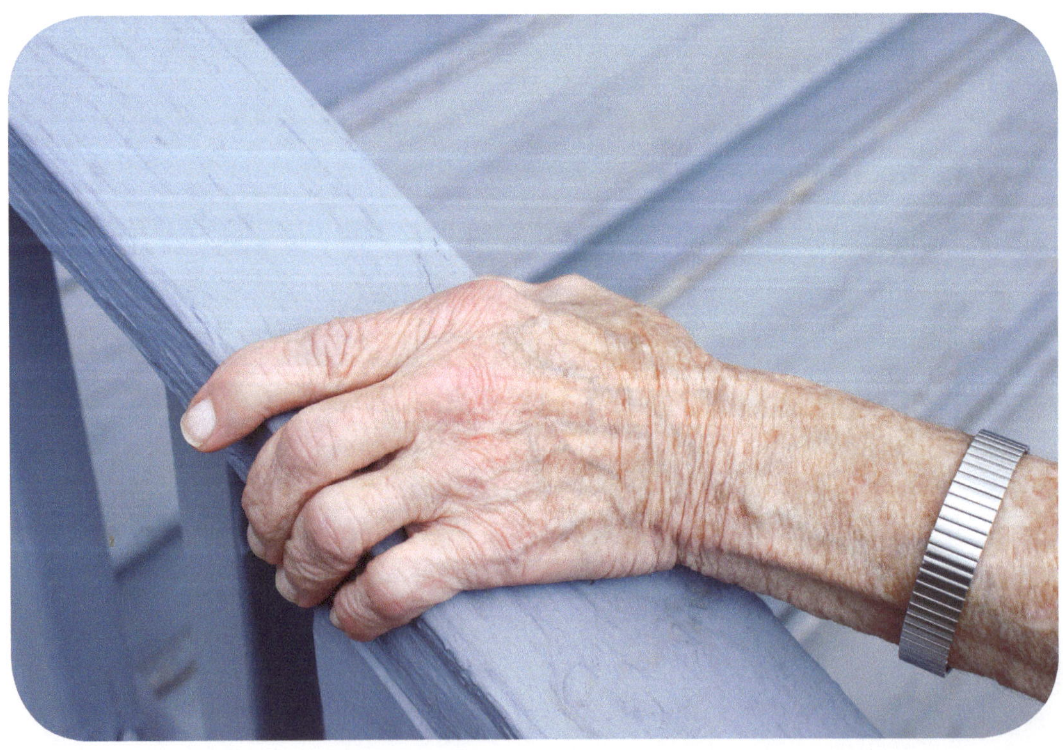

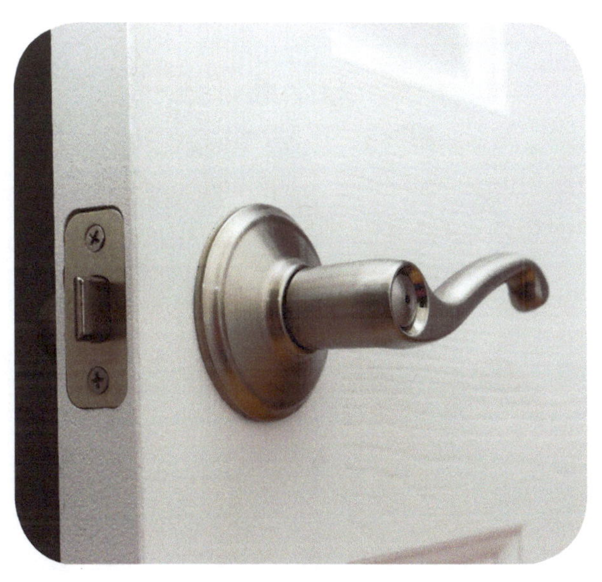

Doorways

If your loved one uses a wheelchair, measure the width to make sure doorways are wide enough. You can remove a door and the molding to make more space if needed. Also have your loved one sit in the wheelchair and reach for the door handle; then change the type of handle if needed. (Knobs are hardest; lever-type handles are easiest.)

Lights, Mirrors, Glass

Check hallways, rooms and closets to make sure they're well lit with no glare or shadows. Add night lights in bathrooms and bedrooms. Good lighting can prevent accidents.

Check your mirrors. Wall-mounted, movable mirrors or hand mirrors can be helpful to those with vision problems or in wheelchairs. Mount mirrors at eye-level for the person sitting in the wheelchair. Put decals, stickers or tape on glass windows and doors to keep those with poor vision from running into them.

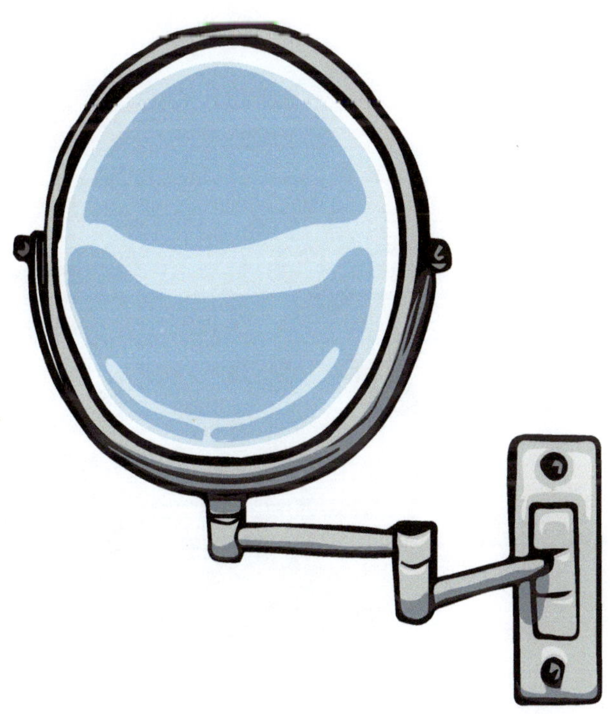

Living Room

Move or take away furniture so there are clear paths to chairs, sofas, TV, etc. Make sure reading areas are well lit. If furniture is too low, put wooden blocks under the legs to raise it up. Make sure it's steady. If cushions are too soft, put boards under them or put another cushion on top.

Bedroom

In the bedroom, the idea is to keep things handy. Make sure there is a bedside table for tissues, toiletries, water, a small bell to call you and anything else your loved one might need.   Place the table on his stronger side. Put a lamp on the table with a switch that is easy for your loved one to work. If needed, adjust the height of the bed for wheelchair transfers. Also, make sure there is enough room to get the wheelchair next to the bed. A firm mattress is a must for someone with poor sitting balance. A bedside commode or bedpan may be needed. If not, make sure there is a clear, well lit path to the bathroom.

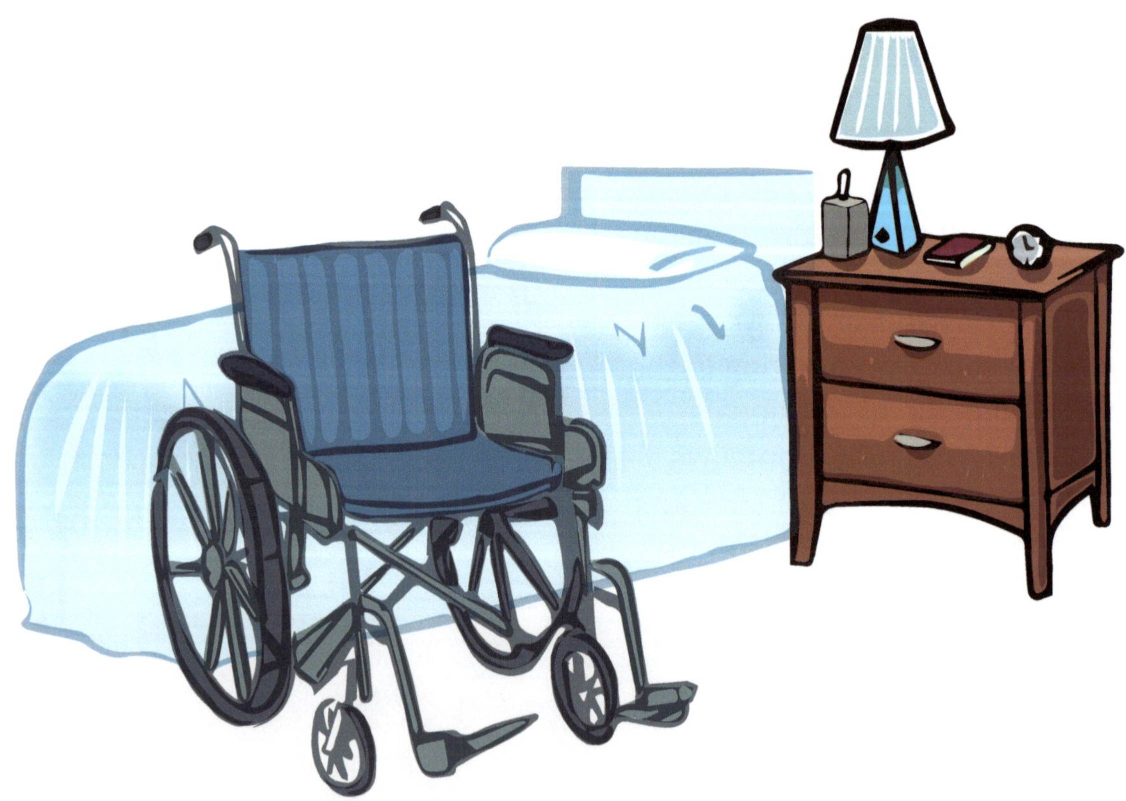

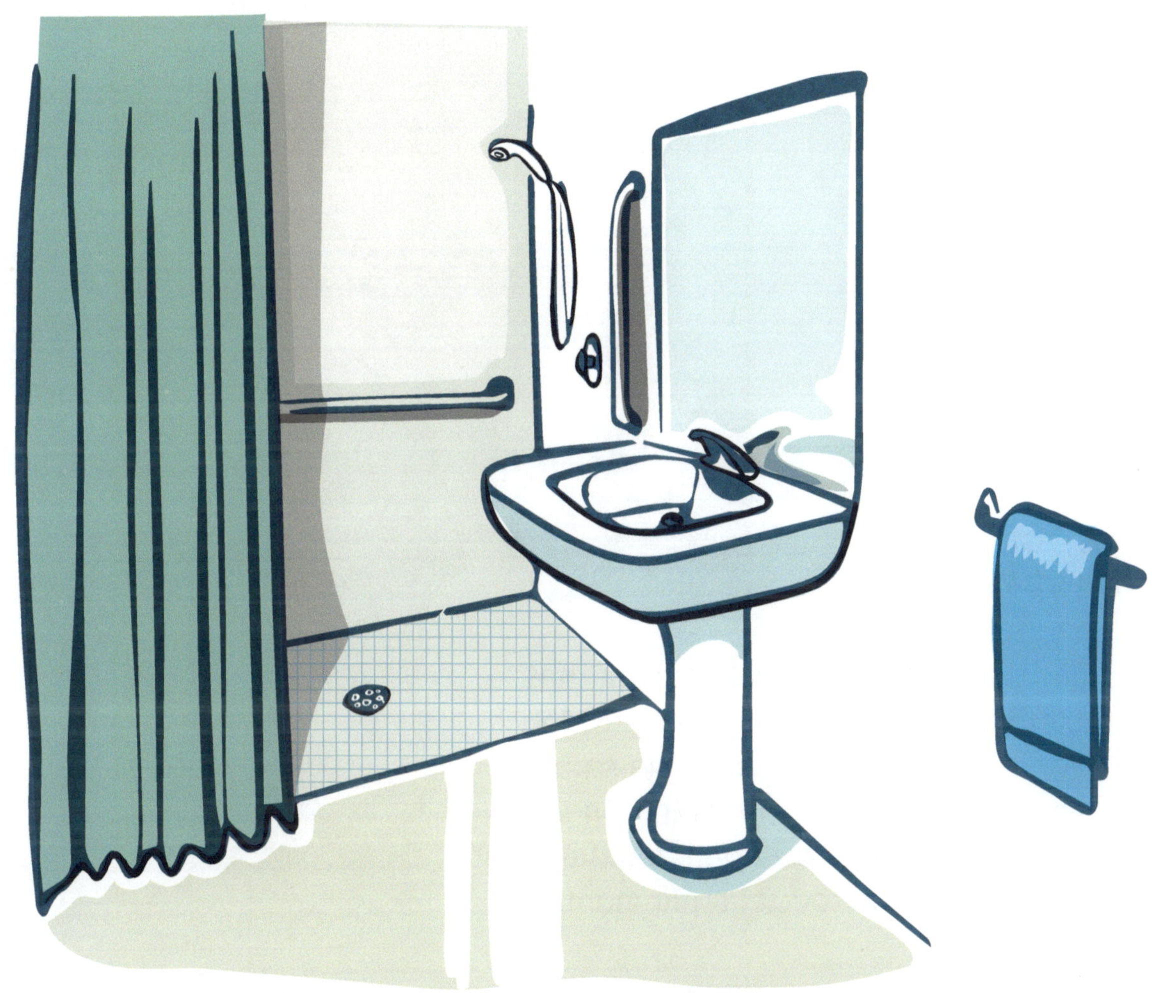

Bathroom

Your loved one will feel better if he can take care of his own bathroom needs without too much help from you. (But make sure you are where you can hear him if he calls.) If you have more than one bathroom, find the one that is easiest to get into and out of.

Then, check with your occupational or physical therapist about ways to make the bathroom work best for your loved one now. For example, toilet seats can be adapted to make them easier to use.

Later, you may want to make more changes to your bathroom. Your therapists can suggest things such as a pedestal type sink or roll in shower, if needed. Check with your therapists before making costly changes, and work with them and the contractor to make a plan that is best for your loved one

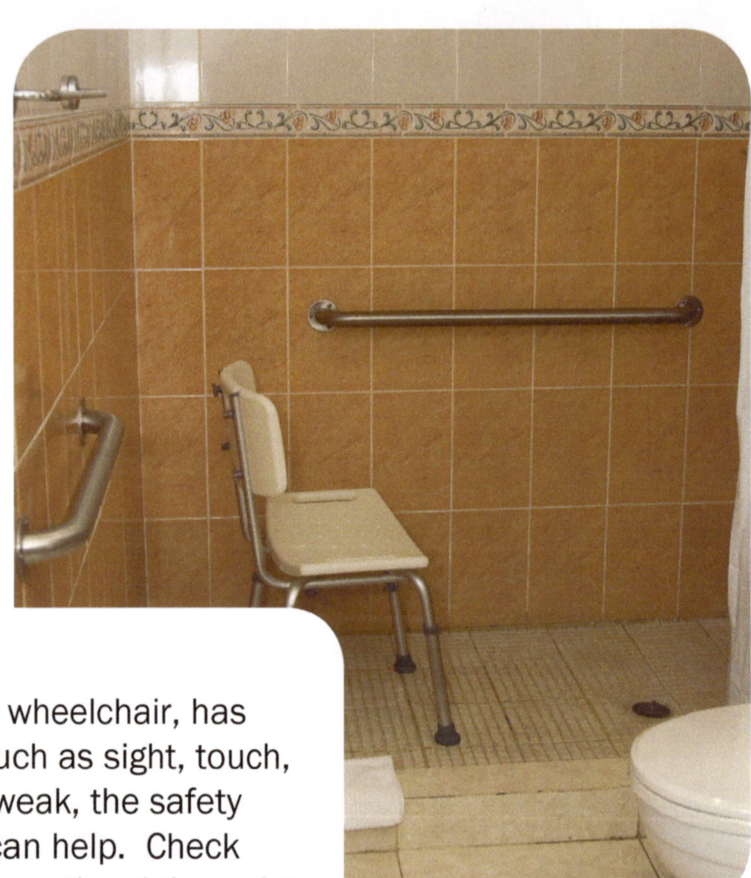

make it safe

If your loved one uses a wheelchair, has problems with senses such as sight, touch, etc. or is unsteady and weak, the safety measures listed below can help. Check with your physical or occupational therapist **before** buying any special equipment.

- Install grab bars by the toilet and in the tub or shower. These must be secured in wall studs.

- Warn loved one not to use soap holders or towel bars as grab bars.

- Use a special tub seat or bench and a nonskid surface in the tub or shower.

- Install a hand-held shower head and large, wing-type faucet handles.

- To avoid burns, check water temperature and cover exposed water pipes with insulation.

- Remove bath mats and floor rugs to prevent falls, or use mats and rugs with rubber backing.

help with grooming

Keep soap, toothbrushes, hair brushes, shampoo, etc. in an easy-to-reach place. Soap on a rope, in a mitt or in pantyhose, prevents it from slipping in the tub or shower. And you can add hooks inside and outside the tub or shower for hanging clothes, wash cloths and hand-held mirrors. If your family member can use only one hand or has a weak arm or hand, check with the occupational therapist about special equipment that might work for him.

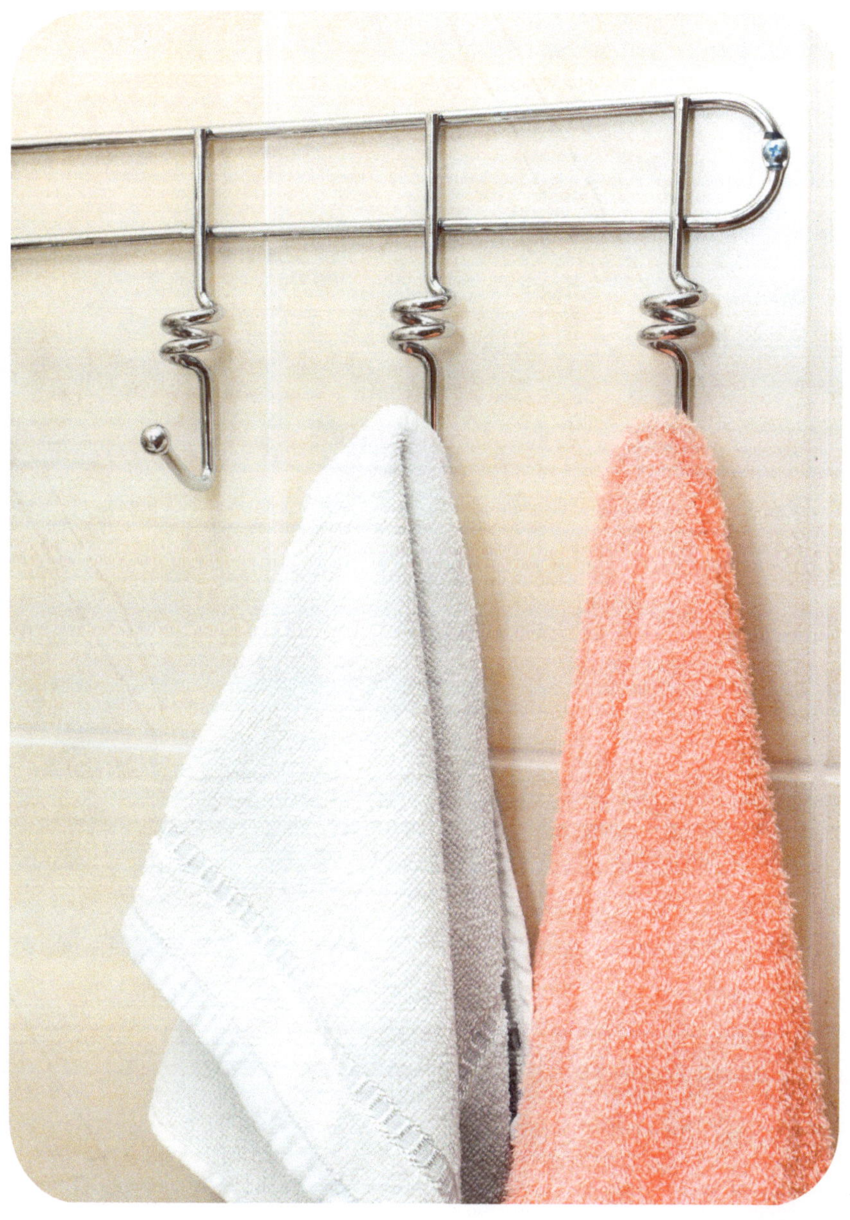

Kitchen

Getting back to kitchen duties may help your loved one feel better. You can work as a team to make a plan for the kitchen. Safety is most important here. Next, think about how to make things easier and even fun! Here are some tips for you and your loved one.

make it safe

- Keep the room well lit.

- Turn pan handles away from edge of stove, and turn burners off when done.

- Pick pans with handles that don't get hot.

- Use mesh screens over pans with hot grease.

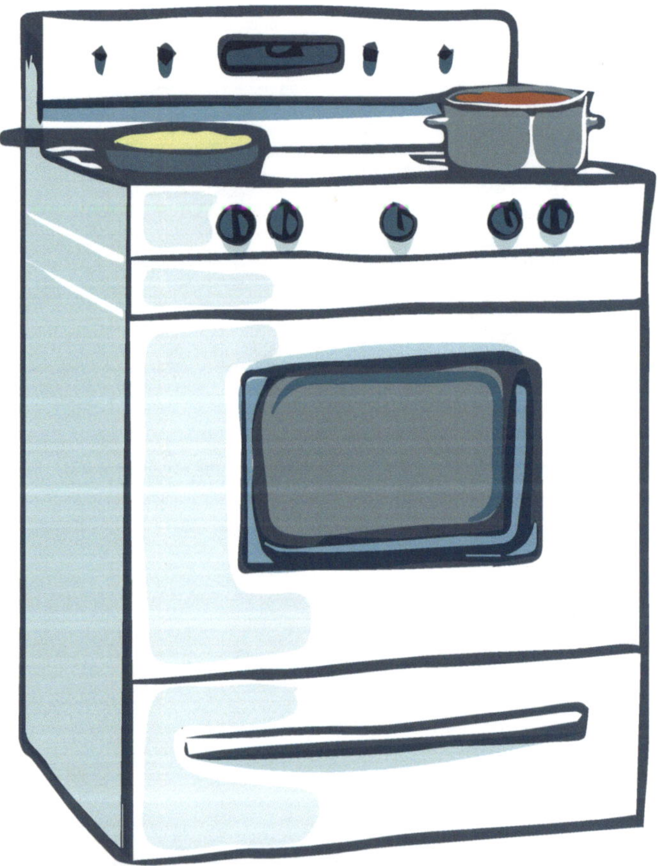

- Keep curtains, blinds, paper towels and
  dish towels away from stove.

- Cover exposed hot water pipes.

- Keep electrical appliances
  away from water.

- Don't wax floors.

- Clean up spills quickly.

- Keep sharp utensils apart
  from others; keep knives in a
  covered rack or knife block.

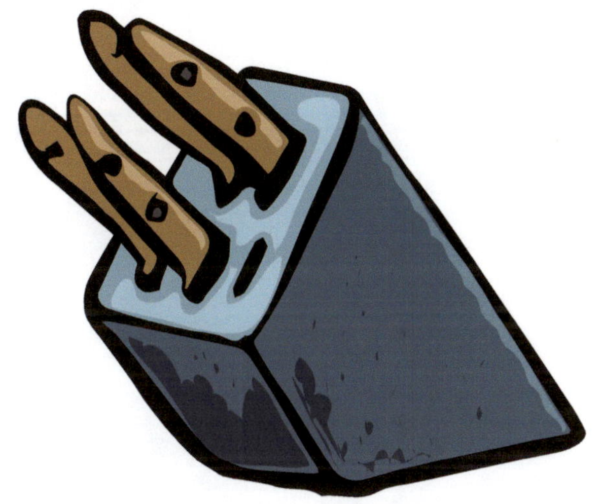

See that your loved one:

- wears nonflammable clothes, oven mitts
  and pot holders

- doesn't wear a plastic apron

- keeps hands dry

- stands to the side when he opens doors (This
  prevents being hit, knocked off balance or having
  to move backwards.)

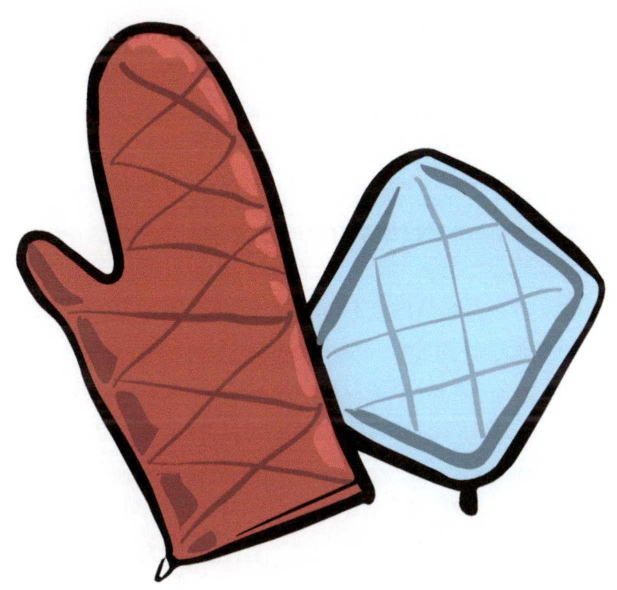

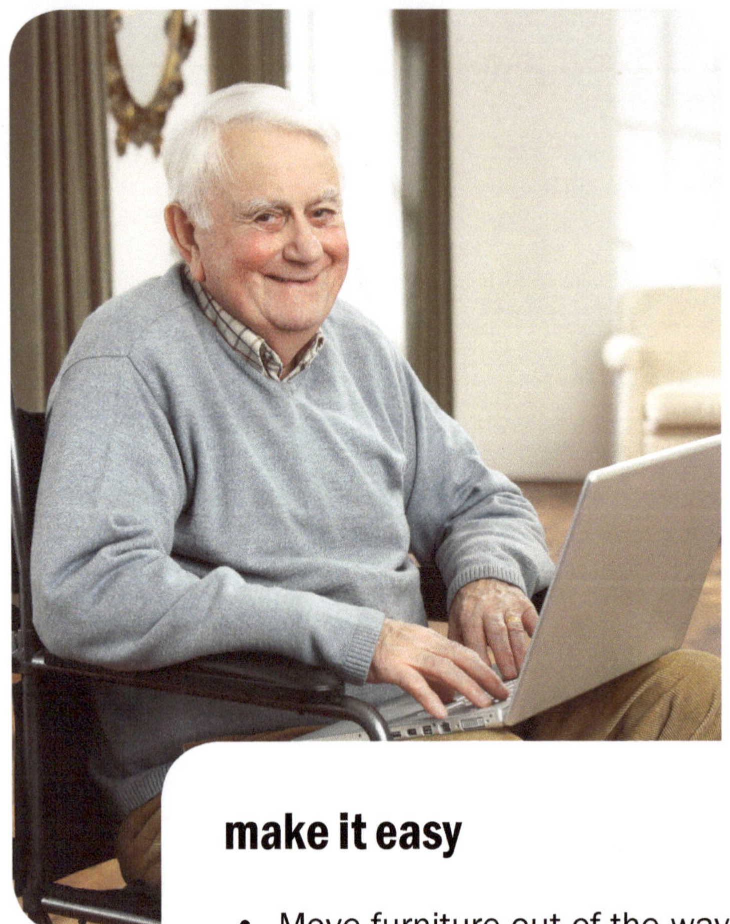

make it easy

- Move furniture out of the way.

- Keep things used often in easy-to-reach places.

- Check with the occupational therapist about special eating tools such as a rocker knife, glass holder, food guard on plate, suction cups for bottom of plate and other gadgets that can help those with use of only one hand or weakness in hand(s).

Have your loved one:

- use a cart on wheels to move things **Do not** lean on cart.

- use apron pockets to carry things that won't spill

- use table, chair or counters as a "bridge" to move things that might spill if using a walker or cane

- sit at the table to work or switch from standing to sitting (if he can't stand for long periods)

All around the house

- Have a telephone with emergency numbers taped to it. A portable phone can be placed in a bag or pouch on a walker or wheelchair.

- Use other calling devices such as a bell, intercom or baby monitor.

- Make sure you have enough fire extinguishers and smoke detectors for your home. Plan a fire escape route.

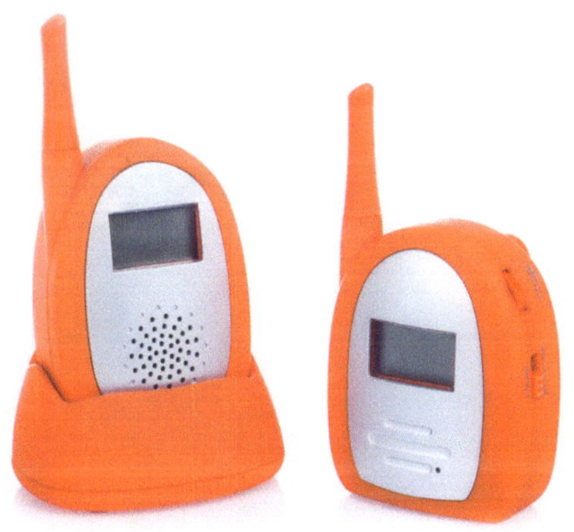

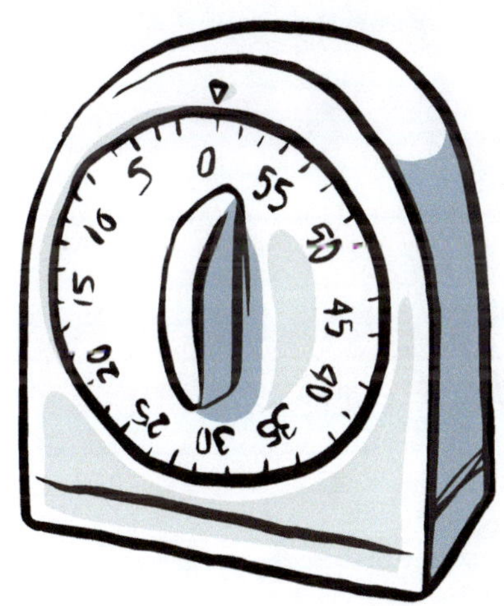

make it easy

- Take your time.

- Make signs for tasks (turn off stove, steps to work microwave).

- Use a kitchen timer to remind your loved one when to do things.

- Ask occupational therapist for other ways to help with memory and thinking problems.

- Relax and think positive thoughts.

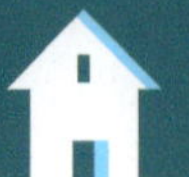

Now you know what changes you need to make in your house and how to make them. You have many ideas about how to keep your loved one safe as he begins to do some things for himself.

As much as you can, include all those living at home in any plans and changes. Things will go smoother, and all of you can benefit from learning to make things safer.

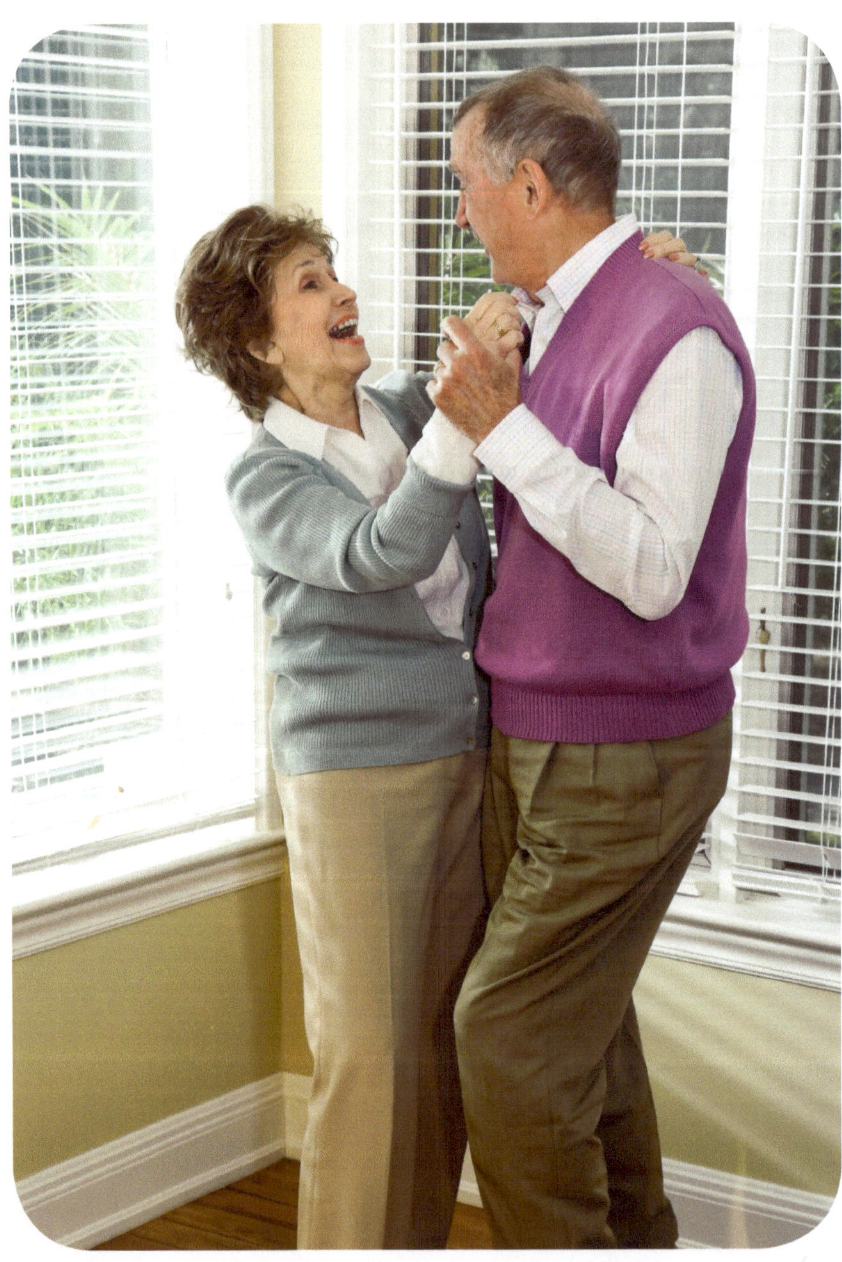

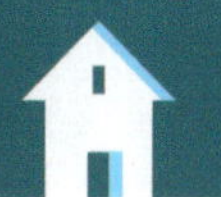

The following list will help you to make your home safer for your loved one. Post near the telephone or on the refrigerator.

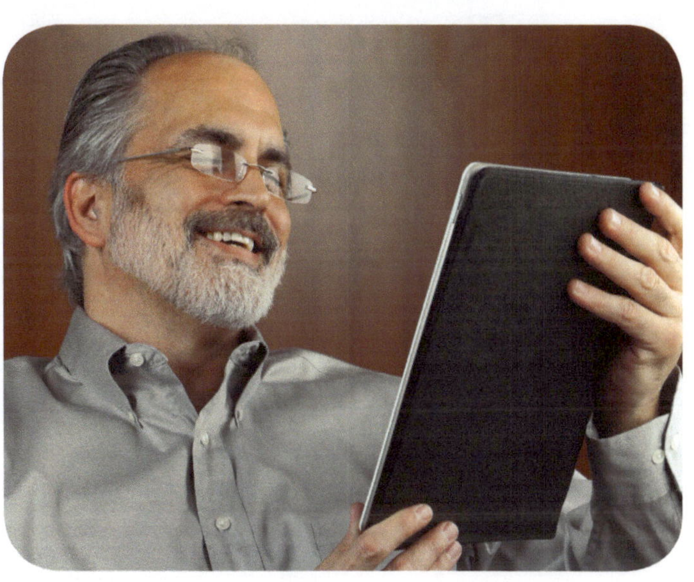

Institute for Human Centered Design
200 Portland Street,
Suite 1
Boston, MA 02114
(617) 695-1225
humancentereddesign.org

National Association for Homecare & Hospice
228 Seventh Street, SE
Washington, DC 20003
(202) 547-7424
nahc.org

National Rehabilitation Information Center
8400 Corporate Drive,
Suite 500
Landover, MD 20785
(800)346-2742
naric.com

Well Spouse Association
63 West Main Street, Suite H
Freehold, NJ 07728
800-838-0879
wellspouse.org

Salmen, John P.S.
The Do-able Renewable Home. Washington, DC: American Association of Retired Persons, 1993. User friendly manual with illustrations and resources for adapting your home for someone with physical limitations is available when you Google "The Do-able Renewable Home".

American Association of Retired Persons
601 E Street NW
Washington, DC 20049
(888) 687-2277
aarp.org

Outside checklist

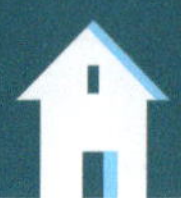

	OK	Not OK	Changes I Need To Make
Parking			
Walkways			
Doors			
Ramp			
Lighting			
Handrails			

Inside checklist

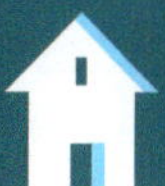

	OK	Not OK	Changes I Need To Make
Flooring			
Furniture			
Stairs			
Doorways			
Lights, Mirrors, Glass			
Living Room			
Bedroom			
Bathroom			
Kitchen			